T0064811

THE CASE AGAINST MASKS

THE CASE AGAINST MASKS

Ten Reasons Why Mask Use Should be Limited

BY DR. JUDY A. MIKOVITS AND KENT HECKENLIVELY, JD

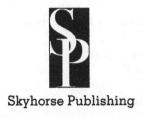

Skyhorse Publishing

Skyhorse Publishing books may be purchased in bulk at special discounts for
sales promotion, corporate gifts, fund-raising, or educational purposes. Special
editions can also be created to specifications. For details, contact the Special Sales
Department, Skyhorse Publishing, 307 West 36th Street, 11th Floor, New York, NY
10018 or info@skyhorsepublishing.com.

Skyhorse® and Skyhorse Publishing® are registered trademarks of Skyhorse
Publishing, Inc.®, a Delaware corporation.

Visit our website at www.skyhorsepublishing.com.

10 9 8 7 6

Library of Congress Cataloging-in-Publication Data is available on file.

Cover art and interior illustrations by Ben Garrison

Print ISBN: 978-1-5107-6427-9
Ebook ISBN: 978-1-5107-6428-6

Printed in the United States of America

"In times of universal deceit, telling the truth is a revolutionary act."

—George Orwell

Contents

Introduction

You know you've seen them. Perhaps you've even been one of them. The people who are so terrified of catching a deadly virus they drive alone in their car with a mask on. Or maybe you go for a walk or run outside, soaking up that good sunshine and vitamin D, but you make sure you put on that mask before you step out your front door. Perhaps while outside you see a young couple pushing a toddler in a stroller and notice the toddler has a mask on in addition to the parents.

It's not my intention to make fun of these people. The information we get is so confusing and contradictory that we collectively shrug and say, "Well, better safe than sorry," and put on a mask before heading out the door. Or maybe you even wear it while inside your house, sitting down to watch television with your family.

Suddenly, the world has become a very terrifying place.

However, I don't believe you make the best decisions when you're scared. The reasoning part of your brain becomes overwhelmed with fear and takes action that, when later considered, seems illogical. Before you get too far into this book, I want you to make a conscious effort to reduce your fear level. If that means you are sitting alone in your bedroom and wearing a mask as you read, terrified of the viral particles you imagine that may be floating unseen around you, then keep that mask on. I doubt you will be wearing it when you finish this book.

I want you to calmly and rationally look at the evidence and arguments in this book and come to your own conclusions.

REASON #1

Oxygen is Good for Human Beings and Carbon Dioxide is Bad!

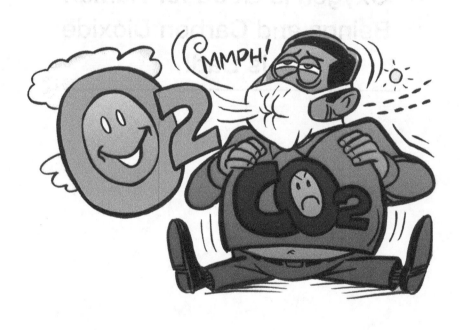

It comes as a surprise to most people to learn oxygen is not the most common gas in our atmosphere. That designation belongs to nitrogen, which according to our most accurate measurements, comprises 78.1 percent of the air we breathe.[1] Nitrogen is an extremely stable gas, and while plants use it for nitrogen fixation (a very critical process for life), it does nothing for us. We breathe it in, and we breathe it out.

By contrast, oxygen makes up only 20.9 percent of our atmosphere and it's where the action is with biological organisms.[2] Oxygen readily engages in chemical reactions and that's why it's critical for life. Carbon dioxide makes up 0.04 percent of our atmosphere.[3] Carbon is also another important element when it comes to creating chemical reactions.

Any science textbook you pick up will tell you that humans need oxygen and give off carbon dioxide as a waste product. If you ever find yourself in a hospital, the nurses may put a blood oximeter on your finger and tell you if your blood oxygen levels are between 95–100 percent you're doing great.[4] If your levels get below 90 percent they'll probably need to take action. Low oxygen levels can be caused by pneumonia, emphysema, smoking, and various heart conditions.

How is it that, while oxygen only makes up 20.9 percent of our atmosphere, it's found at such high concentrations in our blood? The answer is we're oxygen hogs. We desperately need it to power all the chemical and biological reactions necessary for our continued existence and good health. While the world record for holding your breath under water is eleven minutes and thirty-five seconds, it's generally agreed that the average human being will start having trouble if deprived of oxygen for three minutes.[5]

And what about carbon dioxide? It makes up only 0.04 percent of our atmosphere. How much carbon dioxide is in the breath we exhale?

> When inhaling, humans take in approximately 21 percent oxygen, 0.04 percent carbon dioxide and 79 percent nitrogen. On exhalation, humans give off approximately 16 percent oxygen, 4 percent carbon dioxide and 79 percent nitrogen, according to the BBC; only the amount of nitrogen remains constant in the exchange.[6]

In the process of respiration, humans strip out 5 percent of the oxygen from the air, but we cause a hundredfold increase in the amount of carbon dioxide, from 0.04 percent to 4 percent.

OSHA regulations state, "An oxygen deficient atmosphere is an atmosphere that contains less than 19.5 [percent] oxygen, which can cause death."[7] When it's coming out of your mouth, the oxygen level is at 16 percent. Is it a good idea to rebreathe the air you've already exhaled, as inevitably happens in even a cloth mask? It's got lower amounts of oxygen and approximately a hundred times the amount of carbon dioxide.

At what level does carbon dioxide start to become a problem? According to Claire Gillespie, writing at *Health.com*, "It is dangerous in an atmosphere when it is greater than 10[percent]."[8] The level of carbon dioxide in your breath is already 4 percent. How easy is it for the concentration of carbon dioxide in that mask to rise? Gillespie also writes, "When it comes to face masks, we know they're not all made equally. The extent to which a mask could affect CO_2 levels depends on what it's made if, and how tightly it fits."[9]

But isn't the purpose of the mask to control air flow? Isn't that what we're told by people who are supposed to know? Don't we have the innate sense that in order to be effective, the mask must fit tightly, or else what protection does it provide?

In her article, Gillespie references the National Institutes of Health and their warnings about carbon dioxide levels:

> They say that inhaling high levels of carbon dioxide (CO_2) may be life-threatening. Hypercapnia (carbon dioxide toxicity) can also cause headache, vertigo, double-vision, an inability to concentrate, tinnitus (hearing a noise, like a ringing or buzzing, that's not caused by an outside source), seizures, or suffocation due to displacement of air.[10]

There can be life-threatening problems caused by high carbon dioxide levels, but also lower level problems like headaches and vertigo. And this doesn't consider how low oxygen and high carbon dioxide levels can impact other biological processes in the body.

These considerations were detailed in a long letter from four researchers from University College London and published in the *British Medical Journal* in April 2020. Two of their concerns are relevant to our discussion:

> Face masks make breathing more difficult. For people with COPD, face masks are in fact intolerable to wear as they worsen their breathlessness. Moreover, a fraction of carbon dioxide previously exhaled is inhaled at each respiratory cycle. Those two phenomena increase breathing frequency and deepness, and hence they may increase the amount of inhaled and exhaled air. This may worsen the burden of [COVID]-19 if infected people wearing masks spread more contaminated air. This may also worsen the clinical condition of infected people if the enhanced breathing pushes the viral load down into their lungs.[11]

What about people who suffer from COPD (Chronic Obstructive Pulmonary Disease), which is an inflammatory lung condition that affects oxygen flow? What about those who suffer from asthma and other respiratory conditions? Perhaps for most of us a relatively short time of wearing a mask will not cause serious complications. But is that the strategy we want to use if we're trying to maximize our immune function? I'd argue that it is not.

One part of the mask equation is they *do* restrict air flow, and that can never be a result if we want to maintain optimum immune function. But there are other factors which must be considered and may be even more important than restricting air flow:

> While impeding person-to-person transmission is key to limiting the outbreak, so far little importance has been given to the events taking place after a transmission has happened, when innate immunity plays a crucial role. The main purpose of the innate immune system response is to immediately prevent the spread and movement of foreign pathogens throughout the body.
>
> The innate immunity's efficacy is highly dependent on the viral load. If face masks determine a humid habitat where the SARS-CoV-2 can remain active due to the water vapor continuously provided by breathing and captured by the mask fabric, they determine an increase in viral load and therefore they can cause a defeat of the innate immunity and an increase in infections.[12]

Our immune system is designed to limit the spread of pathogens to which we are exposed. One of the main factors in how well our immune system works is what kind of stressors are happening to us. Lack of oxygen can lower the functioning of the immune system. So can stress. If we are in a fearful state, and do not have good personal relations with other people, it negatively affects the functioning of our immune system. It's difficult to escape the conclusion that everything that's being done in the public arena and by our media outlets is crippling the proper working of our immune system.

In the conclusion of their letter to the *British Medical Journal* the authors wrote:

[W]e believe that the context of the current [COVID]-19 pandemic is very different from that of the "parachutes for jumping out of airplanes," in which the dynamics of harm and prevention are easy to define and even to quantify without the need of research studies. It is necessary to quantify the complex interactions that may well be operating between positive and negative effects of wearing surgical masks at population level. It is not time to act without evidence.[13]

The COVID-19 pandemic requires our very best thinking, free of fear and anger. Well-intentioned people can make terrible mistakes. We need to take the emotion out of our analysis and use the available evidence and logical thinking to determine the best course of action.

REASON #2

How Does SARS-CoV-2 Spread?

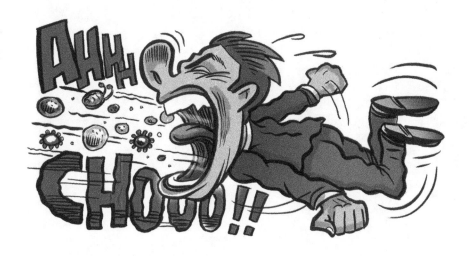

What do we know about how the SARS-CoV-2 virus spreads? Like many questions asked in this book, we may not find a definitive answer. The studies have simply not been done in this early stage of knowledge of a novel virus. But we have some trends which seem to point us in the right direction. While I believe most public health organizations, the World Health Organization (WHO), and the Centers for Disease Control (CDC) have lost significant credibility during this outbreak, I still think it's worthwhile to start with their reporting. We may later find evidence that disagrees with these findings, but let's start with them first.

As detailed in *Guidance on Preparing Workplaces for COVID-19,* produced by the US Department of Labor, Occupational Safety, and Health Administration, "According to the CDC, symptoms of COVID-19 may appear in as few as [two] days or as long as [fourteen] days after exposure."[14] When the lockdown of 2020 first began, it was assumed it would last maybe two or three weeks, so that the curve of the epidemic could be "flattened." As those few weeks lengthened into months, many suspected other agendas were in play. One of the attractive aspects of science is its ability to predict what will happen, given a certain scenario, such as when baking soda and vinegar are mixed together, gas bubbles will be created. It may be in matters of public health that predictions are of limited use, but many feel such shortcomings should have been explained much earlier. In quoting the CDC, the document from the Department of Labor explains:

The virus is thought to spread mainly from person to person, including:

- Between people who are in close contact with one another (within [six] feet).

- Through respiratory droplets produced when an infected person coughs or sneezes. These droplets can land in the mouths or noses of people who are nearby or possibly be inhaled into the lungs.

It may be possible that a person can get COVID-19 by touching a surface or object that has SARS-CoV-2 on it and then touching their own mouth, nose, or possibly their eyes, but this is not thought to be the primary way the virus spreads.

People are thought to be most contagious when they are most symptomatic (i.e., experiencing fever, cough, and/or shortness of breath). Some spread might be possible before people show symptoms; there have been reports of this type of asymptomatic transmission with this new coronavirus, but this is also not thought to be the main way the virus spreads.[15]

The evidence is strong that the virus can spread between people who are in close contact with each other when an infected person coughs or sneezes. Pretty clear, right? Stay away from an infected person. I'll go one step further. Quarantine them. Fourteen days. Fifteen days if you want to be safe. Let the rest of us live our lives and go to work, school, and church.

What's less clear is whether you can be infected by SARS-CoV-2 which contaminated a surface. There was a flurry of discussion in May 2020 on the question of how long SARS-CoV-2 might live on a surface. However, the question is not how long it might live on a surface. The question is how infectious that virus from a surface might be. Remember, the amount of virus to which a person is exposed is also critical. One allied solider on D-Day couldn't liberate Europe, but a half million might be a good start. It's the same with viral load. This was from a *USA Today* article in late May 2020:

Two major findings published within weeks of each other were crucial in shaping what we thought we knew about coronavirus on surfaces.

A study published in the *New England Journal of Medicine* found that viable coronavirus could live on some surfaces, such as plastic and stainless steel, for three days, while surviving for up to [twenty-four] hours on cardboard.

Two weeks after the finding, a CDC report said that genetic material from coronavirus was found on surfaces in the *Diamond Princess* cruise ship [seventeen] days after passengers left their cabins.

Neither of these studies confirmed whether coronavirus spread easily on surfaces. In fact, Joseph Vinetz, a professor of medicine at Yale and infectious disease researcher, said in March that the CDC report "has zero relevance to the ongoing epidemic."[16]

Let's review what we think we know. SARS-CoV-2 viral particles can survive for about a day on cardboard and up to three days on plastic and stainless steel. Why did it survive longer on the *Diamond Princess*? I'm guessing those were areas of the ship that were closed off after the passengers left, remaining warm and humid.

But what were those viral particles not doing while they were on those surfaces? They weren't replicating because there was no organism to host them. That is, the viral particles were becoming weaker. It's important to remember that genetic material is *not* infectious virus. Nor can it be reconstituted to produce infectious virus if it has been in dry air or on a dry surface for more than a few minutes. Yes, you can find it, but it has essentially been disabled.

Further on in the article, another professor from Yale notes, "the process of a person getting infected with COVID-19 by touching a surface requires 'the outer shell of the virus' to remain intact, which remains difficult with proper hand washing and surface cleaning."[17]

From the evidence, it appears the only way you're going to get infected with SARS-CoV-2 (remember, COVID-19 is the disease purportedly caused by SARS-CoV-2) is from somebody who is infected and sick, and they breathe, sneeze, or cough on you. If they aren't sick, you can enjoy all the normal interactions with that person.

My experience comes from interactions with people infected with a much more dangerous and stable RNA virus: HIV. In the twenty-plus years I worked with HIV, I never became infected, and never isolated infectious and transmissible HIV from saliva of *anyone* who wasn't very sick with AIDS (Acquired Immune Deficiency Syndrome). I interacted with them daily from the earliest days of the epidemic when the medical community had no idea what was causing AIDS (then known as Gay Related Immune Disease, GRID), and I was completely safe.

REASON #3

How Effective is a Mask?

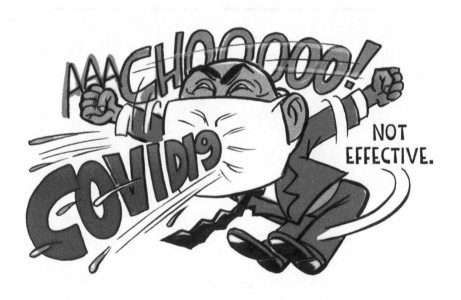

Let's talk about the different types of masks and their effectiveness. Because not all masks are the same and each have their own strengths and weaknesses. The Mayo Clinic put together a short article on this issue.

N95 Masks—It's probably something of a misnomer to call an N95 a mask, when it should more properly be called a respirator, and it's designed to filter out small and large particles. The article says "the mask is designed to block 95 [percent] of very small particles. How small? Micron-sized particles. Viruses are [a thousand] times smaller .... Some N95 masks have valves that make them easier to breathe through. With this type of mask, unfiltered air is released when the wearer exhales."[18] The article details, though, how health care providers have to be trained on how to properly fit the mask to their face and create a proper seal. That provides a certain level of protection, for a time.

However, the N95 masks have additional problems, especially those with a one way-valve, because human beings need to breathe in oxygen and exhale carbon dioxide. "But," the Mayo Clinic continues, "because the valve releases unfiltered air when the wearer breathes out, this type of mask doesn't prevent the wearer from spreading the virus. For this reason, some places have banned them."[19] Yes, you read that correctly. The Mayo Clinic tells you that "some places have banned" N95 respirators. Did you read that in any news accounts? I'm guessing the answer is no.

Surgical masks—These are also called medical masks and are described by the Mayo Clinic as "a loose-fitting disposable mask that protects the wearer's nose and mouth from contact with droplets, splashes and sprays that may contain germs. A surgical mask also filters out large particles in the air. Surgical masks may protect others by reducing exposure to the saliva and respiratory secretions of the mask wearer."[20] I always like to read medical information closely because I'm very pro-science.

Sure, a mask can protect from respiratory droplets. But does it protect from viruses contained in those droplets that are on the mask if the pore size of the mask is a thousand times larger than the virus? Now, instead of protecting, the mask could be increasing risk by concentrating and allowing SARS-CoV-2 and other viruses to remain infectious and transmissible for hours on that mask. What if you wear that mask for a few hours, it's a little damp from your breath, and then you take it off and put in your pocket? That virus now has a nice, warm, and moist environment in which to thrive. Let's just say that the mask does reduce viral transmission and provide some protection from exposure. How much? And what are the other risks?

This is the Mayo Clinic providing this information. I want some data. Why is there no information on how much surgical masks can reduce "exposure to the saliva and respiratory secretions of the mask wearer?" I can have a general feeling this assertion is true, but why is no data offered from which I might draw a conclusion as to the risk/benefit analysis for the wearer? Medical personnel are wearing surgical masks every day in thousands of facilities. How difficult would it be to test this hypothesis? My guess is it would be very simple.

And how does one feel when the Mayo Clinic can't or doesn't choose to provide us with this information?

Cloth masks—The Mayo Clinic article on cloth masks starts out with the general proposition that cloth masks are widely available and can be washed and reused. I think that's an accurate description of reality. They say, "Asking everyone to wear cloth masks can help reduce the spread of the coronavirus by people who have COVID-19, but don't realize it. And countries that required face masks, testing, isolation, and social distancing early in the pandemic seem to have had some success in slowing the spread of the virus."[21]

Let's take apart those few sentences. How can one not realize when one is sick with flu-like symptoms and coughing and sneezing? We are told that countries which implemented "face masks, testing, isolation, and social distancing early in the pandemic seem to have had some success in slowing the spread of the virus." Where is the data to back up this statement? This is what's called anecdotal evidence. It's nothing more than storytelling without evidence to support the claims.

The danger is aptly stated as "people who have COVID-19, but don't realize it." Recall that the incubation period is from two to fourteen days. (Again, we are given little if any data to support this claim for this novel coronavirus, SARS-CoV-2.) One of the guiding principles of science is you test one variable at a time. If you want to find out the effect of sunlight on plant growth, you have one group of plants that receive a normal amount of sunlight and another group that receives no sunlight. Everything else is kept the same—type of soil, temperature, type of plant, and water, to name just a few. The Mayo Clinic lumps four variables together: "face masks, testing, isolation, and social distancing."

We don't know the individual contribution of each factor and we should.

Scientific Research

It's challenging to find high-quality science to answer many questions about masks and I understand why in the absence of good information many might simply say, "better safe than sorry." However, are masks providing benefit or is the wearer at more risk? I still think it's useful to review the limited information we do have.

A 2013 study in the *American Journal of Infection Control* followed ten nurses wearing either an N95 mask or an N95 mask with a surgical mask overlay. In their results section they reported:

Most nurses (90 [percent], n = 9) tolerated wearing respiratory protection for two [twelve]-hour shifts. CO_2 levels increased significantly with baseline measures, especially when comparing an N95 with a surgical mask to only an N95, but changes were not clinically relevant. Perceived exertion; perceived shortness of air; and complaints of headache, lightheadedness, and difficulty communicating also increased over time. Almost one-quarter (22 [percent]) of respirator removals were due to reported discomfort. N95 adjustments increased over time, but other compliance measures did not vary by time. Compliance increased only on day [two], except for adjustments, touching under the N95, and eye touches.[22]

As expected, carbon dioxide levels rose in the nurses from wearing a mask. Nurses complained of shortness of breath, headaches, and lightheadedness. Because of the use of masks, nurses were often touching under the mask (where pathogens would likely be collecting), then often touching their eyes, leading to a reinfection by a pathogen through the eyes. All in all, the article doesn't paint a positive picture of long-term usage of what is generally considered to be the most effective face mask.

A study published in the *Journal of Occupational and Environmental Medicine* in 2018 compared nine different types of face masks commonly used in Beijing, China to see how effectively they filtered out pollution particles:

Results: The mean percent penetration for each mask material ranged from 0.26 [percent] to 29 [percent] depending on the flow rate and mask material. In the volunteer tests, the average total inward leakage (TIL) of BC ranged from 3 [percent] to 68 [percent] in the sedentary tests and from 7 [percent] to 66 [percent] in the active tests. Only one mask showed an average TIL of less than 10 [percent] under both test conditions.

> **Conclusions:** Many commercially available masks may not provide adequate protection, primarily due to poor facial fit. Our results indicate that further attention should be given to mask design and providing evidence-based guidance to consumers.[23]

Problems abounded with these commercially available masks, ranging from the number of particles that would make it through the material to the amount of air that would escape, depending on whether a person was sedentary or active.

How effective are masks? There seems to be a simple dichotomy.

The more effective a mask is at blocking normal air flow, the greater the problem with decreased oxygen and increased carbon dioxide a person is likely to have.

The less effective a mask is at blocking normal airflow, the less a case can be made for using it. And we haven't really dealt with what seems to be the main way that the virus spreads, through coughing and sneezing, which spread respiratory droplets.

REASON #4

Six Feet Apart and Wearing a Mask?

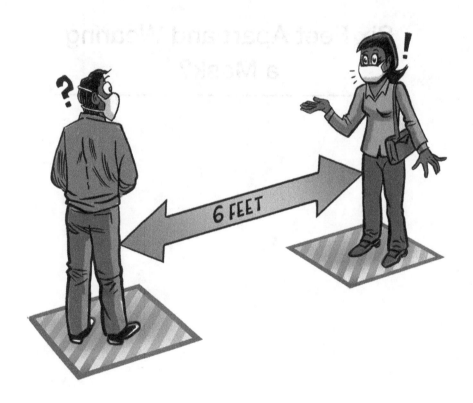

Let's review what we've learned so far. It seems transmission of SARS-CoV-2 is most likely to occur when an infected individual coughs or sneezes on another person. We also understand symptoms may appear within two to fourteen days after exposure. While SARS-CoV-2 particles may live on surfaces for a time, the viral load is likely to be low, and if you touch it after having washed your hands, the chemicals from the soap on your hand will start to break the virus apart. We also understand masks don't really filter as well as you might think because humans need to breathe in oxygen and expel carbon dioxide.

Let's take the worst-case scenario. You're out in public and near somebody who has recently been exposed but has not yet developed symptoms. However, if they haven't yet developed symptoms, they're not likely to be coughing, hacking, or sneezing. But let's say you find yourself next to such a person. What should you do? In that situation, social distancing of three to six feet makes sense. But if you are keeping such social distancing, why do you need a mask? You're already protected. Exposed individuals don't breathe coronaviruses on others. Sick people may cough coronaviruses on others.

In an article for *The Lancet,* published on March 20, 2020, the authors reviewed the conflicting advice given by different countries and organizations regarding face mask usage. For example, in Japan the authors found, "The effectiveness of wearing a face mask to protect yourself from contracting viruses is thought to be limited. If you wear a face mask in confined, badly ventilated spaces, it might help avoid catching droplets emitted from others but if you are in an open-air environment, the use of face masks is not very efficient."[24]

In Hong Kong, the recommendation was, "Surgical masks can prevent transmission of respiratory viruses from people who are ill. It is essential for people who are symptomatic (even if they have mild symptoms) to wear a surgical mask. Wear a surgical mask when taking public transport or staying in crowded places. It is important to wear a mask properly and practice good hand hygiene before wearing and after removing a mask."[25]

In Singapore, it was, "Wear a mask if you have respiratory symptoms, such as a cough or runny nose."[26]

In Germany, the public was told, "There is not enough evidence to prove that wearing a surgical mask significantly reduces a healthy person's risk of becoming infected while wearing it. According to WHO, wearing a mask in situations where it is not recommended to do so can create a false sense of security because it might lead to neglecting fundamental hygiene measures, such as proper hand hygiene."[27]

In the United Kingdom, the recommendation was, "Face masks play a very important role in places such as hospitals, but there is very little evidence of widespread benefit for members of the public."[28]

In the United States, as of March 20, 2020, our lovely citizens were told, "Centers for Disease Control and Prevention does not recommend that people who are well wear a face mask (including respirators) to protect themselves from respiratory diseases, including COVID-19. US Surgeon General urged people on Twitter to stop buying face masks."

Let's talk about what has not taken place since March 20, 2020, when *The Lancet* article was published. Nobody has done any large-scale trials, crunched the data, and shown that masks are effective in preventing the spread of COVID-19. The *Lancet* article observes:

> Evidence that face masks can provide effective protection against respiratory infections in the community is scarce, as acknowledged in recommendations from the UK and Germany. However, face masks are widely used by medical workers as part of droplet precautions when caring for respiratory infections. It would be reasonable to suggest

vulnerable individuals avoid crowded areas and use surgical
face masks rationally when exposed to high-risk areas.[29]

The best-case scenario is that evidence that masks work is
scarce. Common sense would seem to suggest that a strong
case can be made for the use of masks to avoid respiratory
droplets from individuals with respiratory infections. If you
are displaying even mild symptoms, or worry that you might
have been exposed, it's probably a good idea to avoid contact
with other people. If you are not sick, but going into a high-
risk area, like hospitals, nursing homes, or a crowded store,
the temporary use of a mask in those situations could be a
reasonable response.

In an article by *Wired* magazine from April 4, 2020, this
scientific double-standard on masks was addressed, looking
at two studies on whether masking helped prevent influenza
spread. This could likely be a useful stand-in for COVID-19.

> Take, for example a large randomized trial of mask use
> among US college students in the 2006-2007 influenza sea-
> son. The reduction in illness among those wearing face masks
> in that study was not statistically significant. But because
> the research was carried out during what turned out to be a
> mild season for the flu, the trial lacked statistical power for
> that question; there weren't enough sick people for research-
> ers to figure out whether wearing masks improved on hand
> hygiene alone. They also couldn't rule out the possibility that
> students were already infected before the trial began.[30]

Some of the limitations cited by the author are no doubt relevant. But how exactly does a "mild" flu season mean the
entire study is worthless? And they couldn't really compare
the effectiveness of handwashing versus mask wearing? And
finally, they didn't know how many of the students had the
flu before they began? Maybe all these factors were relevant,
or at least suggest more research is needed before conclusions

are drawn, which could be harmful to the most vulnerable in our society.

A study from Australia was even more confusing and leaves a reader wondering about the bias of the researchers:

> Or take another study of the same influenza season, this time in Australia, which found no definitive effect. That one looked at adults living with children who had influenza. Less than half the people randomized into the group of mask wearers reported using them "most or all of the time." In fact, they were often sleeping next to their sick children without them. This bears little resemblance to the question of whether you should wear a mask among strangers at the grocery store in the midst of a pandemic.[31]

It seems to me the results of the experiment, although unintentional, gave two remarkable data sets. The parents who didn't wear the masks often and slept with their children, and those who didn't. Shouldn't that give a strong signal if there was a difference in infection rates of the parents attributable to mask usage?

In addition, the viral load you receive from a sick child with whom one is living in close contact will be much higher than somebody you pass in a supermarket. If there was no effect among family members who live together, why would one expect there would be a greater effect among people who pass each other in public?

The author was arguing in a way which was the exact opposite of logic.

I need to make an additional observation. *Wired* magazine, out of Silicon Valley, has the kind of respect that *TIME* and *Newsweek* enjoyed in a previous generation. Many of today's hottest and smartest young writers contribute articles to the magazine. That's why I was surprised by the argument made by the author that many of our infection precautions are not backed up by good science, but we should follow them anyway.

> It's true that health care workers or other people looking after people sick with [COVID]-19 are exposed to far higher levels of coronavirus than anyone else. In the context of a mask shortage, they obviously have priority claim to access. But that's not to say there isn't support for the use of masks by everyone else. After all, there aren't any clinical trials proving that a [six]-foot social distance prevents infection, as far as we know. (The World Health Organization only recommends a [three]-foot separation.) Nor do clinical trials prove that washing our hands for [twenty] seconds is superior to doing it for [ten] seconds when it comes to limiting the spread of disease in a respiratory disease pandemic.[32]

What's happening to rational thought? I start off agreeing with the initial statement that health care workers are likely to be exposed to high levels of the SARS-CoV-2 virus from infected people, with whom they are in *close* and *sustained* contact. But taking that to the public at large is an enormous leap, especially when one considers the low oxygen and high carbon dioxide levels people will be breathing from their mask. Just because we may want a certain outcome doesn't mean we can rewrite the basic laws of biology.

And that six-foot social distancing rule?

No clinical trials.

The World Health Organization only recommends three feet, even with Ebola when it was discovered in 2014 that some virulent strains could by transmitted by coughing, since Ebola transmits via water droplets, just like SARS-CoV-2.

Feeling confident about the recommendations of your public health officials now?

We don't even know whether it's better to wash your hands for ten or twenty seconds if you're trying to stop a viral outbreak.

The author of the *Wired* article makes an excellent point about how dubious the evidence is for many medical practices, but then seems to ask the question, "If all of our advice isn't really supported by evidence, why are you getting hung up on our advice about masks?" If they want us to follow a certain procedure, and they're telling us it's because that's what the science says, they should at least have the evidence to back it up.

REASON #5

What About Face Seal Leakage and the Backward Jet?

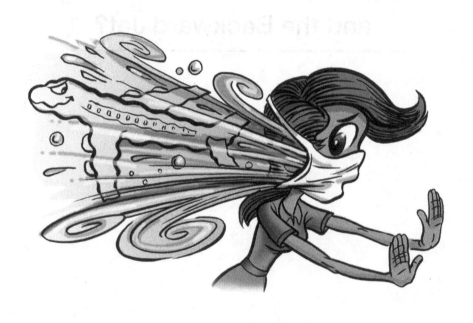

Let's consider the engineering problem with face masks. The intent is to block the flow of air and respiratory droplets from a sneeze or cough from landing on another person or being inhaled. But the force of that sneeze or cough isn't stopped, it's simply redirected. That's basic physics.

Yet it must go *somewhere*.

Like so much of the scientific data about mask usage, there isn't a great deal of good information on this question. However, the research that has been done reveals what might be expected, namely that masks redirect the force of air and respiratory droplets in unexpected ways.

A twelve-thousand-word article on this question by Scottish researchers was submitted to *arVix*, an online digital archive of electronic preprints of scientific papers, on May 19, 2020. The authors wrote:

> The SARS-CoV-2 virus is primarily transmitted through virus-laden fluid particles ejected from the mouth of infected people. In some countries, the public has been asked to use face covers to mitigate the risk of virus transmission—yet, their outward effectiveness is not ascertained. We used a Background Oriented Schlieren technique to investigate the air flow ejected by a person while quietly and heavily breathing, while coughing, and with different face covers.
>
> We found that all face covers without an outlet valve reduce the front flow through jet by more than 90 percent. For the FFP1 and FFP2 masks without exhalation valve, the front through flow does not extend beyond one half and one quarter of a meter, respectively.
>
> Surgical and hand-made masks, and face shields, generate several leakage jets, including intense backward and downward jets that may present major hazards. We also

simulated an aerosol generating procedure (extubation) and we showed that this is a major hazard for clinicians. These results can aid policy makers to make informed decisions and PPE developers to improve their product effectiveness by design.[33]

Let's review some of the important findings of this research. The scientists wanted to investigate what happened to the air flow while people were breathing in a normal manner, while breathing heavily, and while coughing. They found that the masks generally decreased the forward flow of air by 90 percent. I think we can all agree that's a relevant finding and gives us information we didn't have before.

However, the blocking of the forward force of exhaled air means it's being redirected to the sides, down the front of a person, and presumably upwards, which is why many people are finding that their glasses get easily fogged while wearing a mask. These hazards are not fully understood. God designed us to rid ourselves of pathogens as much as possible, but our use of masks is adding an unforeseen obstacle to that design.

It's easy to imagine the redirecting of this exhaled air might be creating viral "hot zones" on a person's face, centered around the eyes, cheeks, and chin underneath the mask. Dr. Russell Blaylock, a well-known writer on medical issues, made these observations in April 2020 on the heightened risks of face masks:

> There is another danger to wearing these masks on a daily basis, especially if worn for several hours. When a person is infected with a respiratory virus, they will expel some of the virus with each breath. If they are wearing a mask, especially an N95 mask or other tightly fitting mask, they will be constantly rebreathing the viruses, raising the concentration of the virus in the lungs and nasal passages. We know that people who have the worst reactions to the coronavirus have the highest concentrations of the virus early on. And this leads to the deadly cytokine storm in a selected number.[34]

So, you really have two choices. One can have a poorly fitting mask which means little protection is being provided the public by the mask doing any filtering of your exhaled air. A tightly fitting mask means you will be rebreathing any virus you do have, increasing the concentration in your nasal passages or your lungs. If your face mask is loosely fitting, you're likely creating viral hot zones on your face. Blaylock continues:

> It gets even more frightening. Newer evidence suggests that in some cases the virus can enter the brain. In most instances it enters the brain by way of the olfactory nerves (smell nerves), which connect directly with the area of the brain dealing with recent memory and memory consolidation. By wearing a mask, the exhaled viruses will not be able to escape and will concentrate in the nasal passages, enter the olfactory nerves and travel to the brain.[35]

God designed us to be as healthy as possible in our natural environment. When exhaling viruses, they would generally be exposed to sunlight or would land on surfaces which were not conducive to their continued existence. Besides concentrating viruses on masks, which we would then touch and handle, raising the level of viruses on our hands, we are also concentrating them on our faces, where they might easily be re-inhaled.

If we understand the greatest danger is from respiratory droplets generated by coughs or sneezes, we should want to know how well masks work when the level of force generated by a cough or sneeze is applied to the material. There may also be unique properties associated with this virus, specifically the size of the viral particle. A letter from South Korean researchers on this question which was published in April 2020 in the *Annals of Internal Medicine* was not reassuring. This is from a *Medpage Today* article on the findings:

A small study from South Korea cast doubt on the ability of surgical or cotton face masks to effectively prevent dissemination of COVID-19 coronavirus from the coughs of infected patients.

Median viral loads did not differ significantly when comparing coughing samples of COVID-19 patients without a mask, with a surgical mask, and with a cloth mask, suggesting these masks were ineffective at filtering SARS-CoV-2, the virus that causes COVID-19, reported Sung-Han Kim, MD, of University of Ulsan College of Medicine in Seoul, South Korea, and colleagues.

In a letter published in *Annals of Internal Medicine*, they cited the size of viral particles as a possible reason for masks' poor ability to filter the virus, despite their effectiveness against other respiratory infections. In particular, prior studies found surgical masks, as well as N95 respirators (which were not tested in the current analysis), help prevent dissemination of influenza virus.[36]

It's understood that in novel situations, such as a new virus, there won't be many studies available, and one will need to look at evidence from similar situations. Masks may provide some protection against influenza, but the size of this virus may make even the comparison to influenza viruses a faulty one.

What is the Actual Risk of Airborne Transmission?

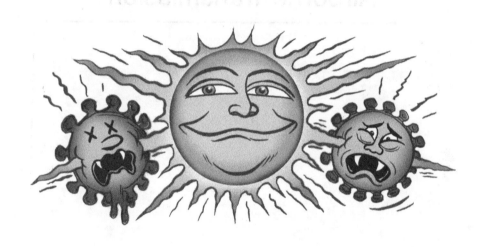

What do we really know about the risk of airborne transmission (not somebody sick who is sneezing or coughing) when you are out and about in your daily life? This might be a classic example of the Sherlock Holmes story in which the biggest clue is the dog that doesn't bark. In other words, let's look at examples of what we do know about the spread of SARS-CoV-2.

One commentator, Jeremy Hammond, a well-known independent journalist, activist, and computer hacker, has written extensively about masks and the conditions under which SARS-CoV-2 can spread, specifically the so-called "super-spreader" events. These unique "super-spreader" events have been used to justify a draconian imposition of universal face-masking.

> For example, in March, [fifty-three] members of a 122-member choir in Washington state were confirmed or presumed to have developed COVID-19 after attending a choir practice. A CDC investigation concluded that transmission occurred through aerosolized viral particles. Dose and duration of exposure is a risk factor for more serious illness, and increased volume increases the amount of aerosols, so an infected person singing or talking loudly in face-to-face contact with others runs the risk of spreading the virus to them.
>
> The spread of the virus by such means requires "unique activities and circumstances"—*like 122 choir members standing in line shoulder-to-shoulder and singing loudly together for a long time.* The CDC drew the conclusion that people in the community setting should maintain six feet of separation and wear cloth coverings *if* social distancing cannot be maintained . . .

Most super-spreader events have occurred indoors, and all have involved groups of people in prolonged close contact with each other.[37]

I have a couple of comments on what is alleged to have happened. Were the people singing in the choir sick and coughing while they were singing? Did the choir members develop COVID-19? Or were they simply demonstrated positive by a test that claimed they'd become infected with SARS-CoV-2? I do not think the accuracy of these tests has been adequately demonstrated at this point. Also, evidence seems to be developing that less than 1 percent of those infected with SARS-CoV-2 will go on to develop symptoms. Much remains to be explained.

But let's assume for a moment that everything as reported is accurate. There is a unique situation posed by more than a hundred people getting together and singing for several hours in a choir. Picture in your mind a typical choir, people standing shoulder-to-shoulder together and singing at a high volume. In that type of situation, different than normal speaking, it is reasonable to believe the virus could spread. For the time being, maybe all choir practices should be suspended. I think that's a rational response to the data.

These questions can be difficult to untangle and were highlighted by an article in *Science*, which posed the question, "Why Do Some Covid-19 Patients Infect Many Others, Whereas Most Don't Spread the Virus at All?" Most importantly, it is absolutely the wrong question to ask if 99 percent of those infected with SARS-CoV-2 are not patients with COVID-19, but healthy people! The most important thing every young scientist learns is to ask the right questions.

Nevertheless, Dr. J. O. Lloyd-Smith, a professor at the University of California, Berkeley, and expert on the role of super-spreaders, explained it this way in the article:

Most of the discussion around the spread of SARS-CoV-2 has concentrated on the average number of new infections caused by each patient. Without social distancing, this reproduction number (R) is about three. But in real life, some people infect many others and others don't spread the disease at all. In fact, the latter is the norm, Lloyd-Smith says: "The consistent pattern is that the most common number is zero. Most people do not transmit."[38]

This is a trusted source saying that most people who have been exposed or infected do not transmit the virus at all. Yes, we need to be concerned about stopping further transmissions of the virus to those most vulnerable of getting COVID-19 from the SARS-CoV-2 infection, so we should use the best available data to achieve that goal.

The *Science* article continued probing the question of what factors go into whether a person is spreading the virus.

Individual patients' characteristics play a role as well. Some people shed far more virus, and for a longer period of time, than others, perhaps because of differences in their immune system or the distribution of virus receptors in the body. A 2019 study of healthy people showed some breathe out more particles than others when they talk. (The volume at which they spoke explained some of the variation.) Singing may release more virus than speaking, which could help explain the choir outbreaks. People's behavior also plays a role. Having many social contacts or not washing your hands makes you more likely to pass on the virus.[39]

This section of the article reinforces many of the main points of this book. Healthy people are not "patients." The immune system of the person is an important factor in the spread of the virus. What things do we know that can improve the functioning of the immune system? Keeping your stress low, getting enough sleep, having good and enjoyable social interactions, getting exercise, eating healthy food, and getting enough of that good vitamin D from sunlight. There's likely to be many genetic and epigenetic (environmental) factors, as well. If you're a loud talker, maybe you want to lower that a bit. Since we know that the presence of soap residue on your hands is likely to break down the virus, hand washing seems to be an important factor.

One of the experts consulted for the *Science* article was Dr. Gwenan Knight of the London School of Hygiene and Tropical Medicine:

> Some situations may be particularly risky. Meatpacking plants are likely vulnerable because many people work closely together in spaces where low temperature helps the virus survive. But it may also be relevant that they tend to be loud places, Knight says. The report about the choir in Washington made her realize that one thing links numerous clusters: They happened in places where people shout or sing. And although Zumba classes have been connected to outbreaks, Pilates classes, which are not as intense, have not, Knight notes. "Maybe slow, gentle breathing is not a risk factor, but heavy, deep, or rapid breathing and shouting is."[40]

The question of temperature and sunlight has rarely come up in public discussions of this virus, but this may account for the general observation that viral outbreaks tend to fade in the warm summer months. However, in late April 2020, a senior official with Homeland Security directly addressed these questions.

> William Bryan, science and technology advisor to the Department of Homeland Security secretary, told reporters at the White House that government scientists had found ultraviolet rays had a potential impact on the pathogen, offering hope that its spread may ease over the summer . . .
>
> It showed that the virus's half-life—the time taken for it to reduce to half its amount—was [eighteen] hours when the temperature was 70–75 degrees Fahrenheit (21–24 degrees Celsius) with 20 percent humidity on a non-porous surface . . . .

But the half-life dropped to six hours when the humidity rose to 80 percent—and to just two minutes when sunlight was added to the equation.[41]

Sunlight under the right conditions can destroy the virus in two minutes. One assumes that a colder temperature, but with sunlight, would take just a little while longer, while a higher temperature would make the process go even faster. Why are we being advised to stay in our houses when the best thing we could do to eradicate the virus would be to go out into the sunlight for a few minutes? In the laboratories where I worked daily with concentrated viral stocks, we decontaminated surfaces continuously by turning on UV lights every night before we left.

Another researcher who was consulted was Dr. Adam Kucharski, also of the London School of Hygiene and Tropical Medicine, who added another factor to the mix.

Timing also plays a role. Emerging evidence suggests COVID-19 patients are most infectious for a short period of time. Entering a high-risk setting in that period may touch off a superspreading event, Kucharski says. Two days later, that person could behave in the same way and you wouldn't see the same outcome."[42]

There seems to be multiple factors that are critical in the spread of SARS-CoV-2 and the development of COVID-19. Different individuals, if infected, will expel different amounts of virus, likely due to the loudness of their speaking or singing, their closeness to other individuals, and the time they're together. Cold temperatures are more likely to support the spread of the virus than warm temperatures, if only by increasing the possibility that an infected person will cough or sneeze. Sunlight is a potent killer of this virus. Another factor may be that even if infected there is a relatively brief time in which a person is more infectious. This time period can be enhanced by cold temperatures or lack of exposure to UV light.

Does universal masking make sense when we consider all these factors? Actually, consideration of these factors suggests universal masking increases the risk of spreading the infection.

What is a Dangerous Situation for the Vulnerable Exposed to SARS-CoV-2 to Develop COVID-19?

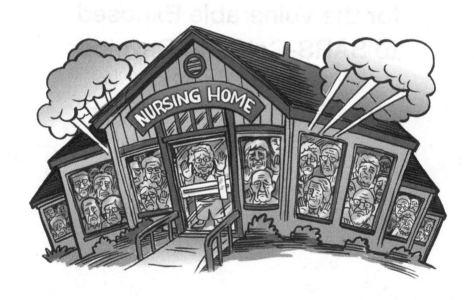

Let's go to what is without doubt the single greatest catastrophe in the SARS-CoV-2 outbreak: the deaths in nursing homes. *Forbes* magazine, in an article from May 26, 2020, reported it this way: "The Most Important Coronavirus Statistic: 42 [percent] of U.S. Deaths are from 0.6 [percent] of the Population." One simple fact is that 42 percent might be too low a number.

> And 42 [percent] could be an undercount. States like New York exclude from their nursing home death tallies those who die in a hospital, even if they were originally infected in a long-term care facility. Outside of New York, more than half of all deaths from COVID-19 are of residents in long-term care facilities.
>
> Prior to last week, Ohio reported that 41 [percent] of COVID deaths were taking place in long-term care facilities. But updated disclosures last Friday, taking deaths prior to April 15 into account, upped that share to 70 [percent].
>
> In Minnesota, 81 [percent] of all COVID-19 deaths are of nursing home and residential care home residents. The region from the eastern seaboard from Virginia to New Hampshire has been especially hard-hit.[43]

When one looks at data the question must always be asked concerning its reliability. Ohio had reported 41 percent of their deaths were from long-term care facilities, but when they checked the numbers, they jumped to 70 percent. In Minnesota the numbers were even more alarming, with 81 percent of the deaths coming from nursing homes and similar arrangements. If the numbers were thoroughly checked through the country, would we see a similar pattern?

A question which should be asked in those states which sent infected residents back into nursing homes is: Did this action contribute to the death toll? This is not a political question, it's a scientific one. We need to know the answer to this question, regardless of the political party of the persons who made the decision. The political risk, falling mostly on governors in democratic states, is whether that will lead to a loss in the next election. But that cannot be our concern. We need to know how many senior citizens died because of the bad decisions of politicians. *Forbes* continued:

> The tragedy is that it didn't have to be this way. On March 17, as the pandemic was just beginning to accelerate, Stanford epidemiologist John Ioannidis warned that "even some so-called mild or common-cold-type coronaviruses have been known for decades [to] have case fatality rates as high as 8 [percent] when they infect people in nursing homes." Ioannidis was ignored.
>
> Instead, states like New York, New Jersey, and Michigan actually ordered nursing homes to accept patients with active COVID-19 infections who were being discharged from hospitals.
>
> The most charitable interpretation of these orders is that they were designed to ensure that states would not overcrowd their ICUs. But well after hospitalizations peaked, governors like New York's Andrew Cuomo were doubling down on their mandates.[44]

It seems relatively clear from the *Forbes* article that even the common-cold-type coronaviruses (many don't realize that the common cold is a coronavirus) can cause high mortality in nursing homes. Given this prior knowledge, it seems incomprehensible that politicians such as New York Governor Andrew Cuomo would order nursing homes to accept COVID-19 patients who were being dismissed from hospitals.

If we understand how the numbers are skewed toward the older population in nursing homes, what does that mean for the rest of us?

There is one silver lining—or perhaps bronze lining—to the COVID long-term care tragedy. The fact that nearly half of all COVID-19 deaths have occurred in long-term care facilities means that the 99.4 percent of the country that *doesn't* live in those places is roughly half as likely to die of the disease than we previously thought.

Many European countries have struggled with the same nursing home problems that we have. But based on the mounting evidence that serious illness from COVID-19 is concentrated in the elderly, Switzerland and Germany have reopened their primary and secondary schools. Sweden, for the most part, never closed them to begin with. Germany has kept most of its factories in operation, and Sweden's restaurants remain open.[45]

We can more fully appreciate that most deaths are among the elderly, especially from nursing homes in which they are grouped together. Sending COVID-19 patients discharged from hospitals back to their nursing homes seems to have been a disaster. Now, can we get even greater clarity on those who are likely to die from COVID-19?

An article posted on the Microsoft Network on June 16, 2020 from *Statista*, a German online portal for statistics, reviewed the data from the Centers for Disease Control.

The CDC has reported that coronavirus patients with underlying health conditions are hospitalized at a rate six times as often as healthy individuals while they die [twelve] times as often. The data focuses on 1.32 million laboratory-confirmed COVID-19 cases between January 22 and May 30 across the U.S. and it compared hospitalization rates, ICU admission rates and death rates for patients both with and without underlying conditions. The most common

underlying medical conditions reported in American coronavirus patients are heart disease (32.2 percent), diabetes
(30.2 percent), and chronic lung disease (17.5 percent.)[46]

When the data are shown to a person, the fear can begin
to lessen. Facts are important. Hearsay and propaganda can
be deadly, as demonstrated by these examples. Patients with
underlying health conditions are six times more likely to be
hospitalized and twelve times more likely to die than those
with no underlying health conditions. The most common
underlying health conditions that contribute to COVID-19
mortality are heart disease, diabetes, and chronic lung disease (mostly COPD).

Some specific numbers are then provided in the article.
Now, remember, this is for those individuals who contract
the coronavirus, not simply the public at large.

> The CDC reported that the hospitalization rate for otherwise
> healthy coronavirus patients in the U.S. is 7.6 percent while
> it is 45.4 percent for those with underlying conditions. The
> gulf in the ICU admission rate is also glaring, as is the death
> rate. 1.6 percent of the seemingly healthy patients without
> any underlying health conditions died during the period of
> the analysis compared to 19.5 percent of patients who did
> have underlying medical concerns.[47]

I'm sorry, there's no such thing as a "healthy" patient.
That's an oxymoron, like jumbo shrimp or alone together.
Nevertheless, the risk factors start to come into focus.

Healthy people who are infected with coronavirus have a
7.6 percent chance of needing to be hospitalized, while having a 92.4 percent likelihood of not being hospitalized.

People with underlying conditions have a 45.4 percent
chance of hospitalization for coronavirus, but only a 54.6 percent chance of avoiding hospitalization.

Healthy people who get SARS-CoV-2 infection have a 1.6
percent chance of dying and a 98.4 percent chance of survival.

(More recent data suggests the actual number is a 0.04 per-cent chance of dying and a 99.96 percent chance of survival.)

People with underlying conditions have a 19.5 percent chance of dying from SARS-CoV-2 and an 80.5 percent chance of surviving.

Can a Mask Become a Virus Trap?

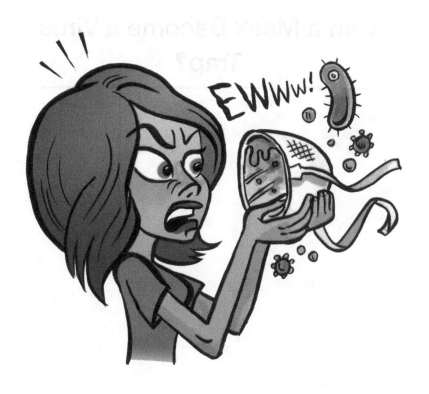

We've spent a good deal of time talking about whether masks will protect people who wear them, or others around them. Now it's time to talk specifically about the mask and the condition it is in after several hours of being on a person's face, which we touched upon briefly in the early chapters. An article in *Science Daily* from January 2017 accurately summed up the problem:

> Airborne pathogens like influenza are transmitted in aerosol droplets when we cough or sneeze. The masks may well trap the virus-laden droplets, but the virus is still infectious on the mask. Merely handling the mask opens up new avenues for infection. Even respirators designed to protect individuals from viral aerosols have the same shortcoming—viruses trapped in respirators still pose risks for infection and transmission.[48]

If we assume the mask has prevented some viral particles from escaping, even from a sneeze or cough, we now have a highly contaminated item which individuals are treating as if it is free from danger.

Most agree that the N95 respirators provide the highest level of protection, but in their own publication the Centers for Disease Control (CDC) detail the potential problems of them becoming a virus trap:

> Respiratory pathogens on the respirator surface can potentially be transferred by touch to the wearer's hands and thus risk causing infection through subsequent touching of the mucous membranes of the face (i.e., self-inoculation). While studies have shown that some respiratory pathogens remain infectious on respirator surfaces for extended periods of time,

> in microbial transfer and re-aerosolization studies more than
> 99.8 [percent] have remained trapped on the respirator after
> handling or following simulated cough or sneeze.[49]

By virtue of the mask being over a person's face for the entire
day, the mask itself has become a highly contaminated surface, especially on the inside portion of the mask. A simple
reach inside the mask, perhaps to scratch an itch on the cheek
or nose, now makes it likely that the person's finger is loaded
with viruses. A wipe of the eyes means the virus has been
transferred to the watery surface of the eye, where it now has
a clear path to the brain.

But let's imagine transmission might come from another
source, the person who is not wearing the mask. The exterior
portion of the mask is supposed to provide some filtering of
respiratory droplets from a person coughing or sneezing, or
aerosolized particles drifting through the air. That means that
the exterior, outward facing part of the mask is now contaminated. The CDC publication also addresses this problem:

> Respirators might also become contaminated with other
> pathogens acquired from patients who are co-infected with
> common healthcare pathogens that have prolonged environ-
> mental survival (e.g., methicillin-resistant Staphylococcus
> aureas, vancomycin-resistant enterococci, Clostridium diffi-
> cile, norovirus, etc.). These organisms could then contam-
> inate the hands of the wearer, and in turn be transmitted
> via self-inoculation or to others via direct or indirect contact
> transmission.[50]

To recap the potential problems, the inside portion of the
mask may become contaminated with viruses that are being
exhaled by the wearer and then kept viable by the continued exhalation of warm, moist air. The exterior portion of
the mask may also become contaminated by persons other
than the wearer, who have other pathogens, and may be

coughing or sneezing or ejecting aerosolized particles containing viruses.

Any touching of the mask, even inadvertent, is likely to transfer these viruses to the fingers of the person wearing the mask.

The Myth of Asymptomatic Carriers

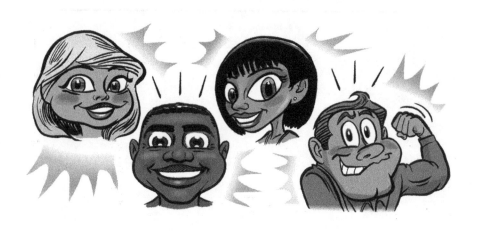

What does it mean to be an asymptomatic carrier of SARS-CoV-2? Probably no other question in the COVID-19 debate has been the subject of more confusion. Let's start simply. If you are "asymptomatic," that means you have no symptoms, either fever, coughing, sneezing, or hacking, which might put others at risk for respiratory droplets. It's probably more accurate to say one is "pre-symptomatic," meaning that they might develop in the two to fourteen-day latency period observed in COVID-19.

However, there are no "asymptomatic" carriers, meaning infected individuals who are carrying around the virus unknowingly for weeks, months, or years. If you are exposed to coronavirus and have even a mild reaction, your immune system has now produced anti-bodies to the virus and you have cleared the virus.

On June 8, 2020, the World Health Organization (WHO) addressed this issue and said:

> "It still seems to be rare that an asymptomatic person actually transmits onward," epidemiologist Maria Van Kerkhove, WHO's technical lead for the coronavirus said. "We have a number of reports from countries who are doing very detailed contacts, and they're not finding secondary transmission onward. It's very rare."[31]

But that wasn't the end of the story. After receiving a great deal of criticism for her statement, the WHO issued a clarification the following day.

> The WHO maintains that what was said was not in error, but perhaps the word asymptomatic was interpreted too broadly,

to include people who may not yet be showing symptoms (pre-symptomatic), or people with very mild illnesses.[52]

In order to provide an example so that it might be clearer to people the actual type of risk they were attempting to describe, WHO said:

> One telling example: in May, officials in Seoul, South Korea traced as many as [forty] coronavirus cases back to nightclubs after one man visited three of them, and later tested positive for COVID-19, the disease caused by the coronavirus.
>
> "That means you could be in the restaurant, feeling perfectly well, and start to get a fever," Ryan said. "You didn't think you'd need to stay home, but that's the moment at which your viral load could be actually quite high . . . It's because the disease can spread at that moment that the disease is so contagious. That's why it's spread around the world in such an uncontained way."[53]

It is understandable one might think to wear a mask because of the fear that somebody around you might suddenly develop symptoms, at which point they are likely to be highly contagious, when this situation has never in human history proved true, even in the SARS and MERS pandemics of 2001 and 2009 respectively. That said, even with mild social distancing, and not hanging around in nightclubs or choirs, one should be able to avoid such risks and limit the spread, just as likely occurred in those pandemics.

A study by Japanese researchers and Harvard University was conducted on patients from the *Diamond Princess* cruise ship to try and tease out the risk of the so-called "asymptomatic patients." Despite having a population of 3,711 people and 634 coming down with the virus, the study concluded:

> Currently, there is no clear evidence that COVID-19 asymp-
> tomatic persons can transmit SARS-CoV-2, but there is
> accumulating evidence indicating that a substantial fraction
> of SARS-CoV-2 infected individuals are asymptomatic.[54]

One must always be open to possibilities revealed by new information, but from what has been demonstrated so far, the risk of transmission from an "asymptomatic carrier" (however one might choose to define that), appears extremely small. Again, when they say "asymptomatic" they mean an individual who is "pre-symptomatic" or who may have only mild symptoms which might easily be missed.

Perhaps one of the most definitive analyses of the mask issue was conducted in late May 2020 by the prestigious *New England Journal of Medicine.*

> We know that wearing a mask outside health care facilities
> offers little, if any, protection from infection. Public health
> authorities define a significant exposure to [COVID]-19 as
> face-to-face contact within [six] feet with a patient with
> symptomatic [COVID]-19 that is sustained for at least a
> few minutes (and some say more than [ten] minutes or even
> [thirty] minutes). The chance of catching [COVID]-19 from
> a passing interaction in a public space is therefore minimal.
> In many cases, the desire for widespread masking is a reflex-
> ive reaction to anxiety over the pandemic.[55]

These authors are destroying the entire rationale for widespread masking. Their understanding of the warnings from public health officials is that you are in danger if you have face to face contact with a "symptomatic" COVID-19 patient for at least a few minutes, if not anywhere from ten to thirty minutes. Your risk of contracting COVID-19 from a brief interaction in a public place is "minimal." The call for widespread masking is best understood as a "reflexive reaction to anxiety over the pandemic."

Remember what we said about "fear" overriding your rational mind? That's what we're getting from so many of our politicians, public health officials, and celebrities like Joy Behar who claim to be driving around their cities and "mask-shaming" those who aren't wearing their masks.[56] Fear over facts. I'm pleased that the researchers tackle these questions in such an honest manner, but it also seems that in their interpretation of the data, they succumb to some of the anxiety.

> There may be additional benefits to broad masking policies that extend beyond their technical contribution to reducing pathogen transmission. Masks are visible reminders of an otherwise invisible yet widely prevalent pathogen and may remind people of the importance of social distancing and other infection-control measures.
>
> It is also clear that masks serve symbolic roles. Masks are not only tools, they are also talismans that may help increase health care workers' perceived sense of safety, well-being, and trust in the hospitals. Although such reactions might not be strictly logical, we are all subject to fear and anxiety, especially during times of crisis. One might argue that fear and anxiety are better countered with data and education than with a marginally beneficial mask, particularly in light of the worldwide mask shortage, but it is difficult to get clinicians to hear this message in the heat of the current crisis.[57]

Call me crazy, but I'll take data and education over a "talisman" every day. My coauthor, Kent, enjoys fantasy movies like Harry Potter as much as anybody, but magical talismans are not what either of us would deploy against a purported causative agent, SARS-CoV-2 of the deadly disease, COVID-19. And while we understand medical experts are human, we do expect their training has taught them to suppress their fear and anxiety enough so they can focus on good data and develop a reasonable plan.

If they can't, they should find another profession.

REASON #10

Children Do NOT Need to Wear a Mask to Return to School

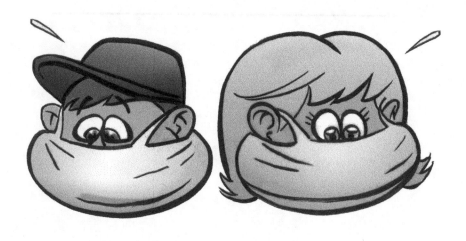

One of the most challenging questions is how to protect our children from developing COVID-19. In some ways, however, they seem to be less in need of protection than the adult population. As stated in an article in *STAT* from June 18, 2020:

> Kids get sick, pass the viruses among themselves, and infect the adults in their lives—teachers, day care attendants, parents, and grandparents. It's not a coincidence that elementary school teachers are often sniffling and sneezing within a month of the start of school, or that flu season often hits in earnest after Thanksgiving or Christmas, when multiple generations share holiday cheer and the occasional germ.
>
> If children play the same role with the SARS-CoV-2 virus, closing schools and restricting the access of children to each other and the older adults in their lives could be important ways to suppress transmission of the new disease. But if they play a less active role, as studies seem to suggest, then the high cost of these restrictions—interrupted education and socialization, stress as parents juggle working from home with child care, lack of access to school meals—aren't warranted by the small benefits gained.[58]

The simple fact seems to be that children are not significantly impacted by COVID-19. If they do contract SARS-CoV-2, few examples of the development of anything more than a mild cold is evident. And even if children do contract SARS-CoV-2, they do not seem to spread the infection.

An article in *Science* magazine attempted to make sense of this mystery, highlighting some of the unexpected findings among children:

For families eager for schools to throw open their doors, the
tale of a [nine]-year-old British boy who caught COVID-
19 in the French Alps in January offers a glimmer of hope.
The youngster, infected by a family friend, suffered only
mild symptoms; he enjoyed ski lessons and attended school
before he was diagnosed. Astonishingly, he did not transmit
the virus to any of [seventy-two] contacts who were tested.
His two siblings didn't become infected, even though other
germs spread readily among them: in the weeks that followed, all three had influenza and a common cold virus.

The story could be a bizarre outlier—or a tantalizing
clue. Several studies of COVID-19 hint that children are less
likely to catch the novel coronavirus, and don't often transmit it to others. A recent survey of the literature couldn't find
a single example of a child under [ten] passing the virus on to
someone else, for example.[59]

To be certain, there are differences between children under
the age of ten and those over, but they don't appear to be
significant. The pattern repeats again and again. If you have
a strong immune system (which is likely to be strongest when
you are young), the virus does not seem to present significant
risk. Also, the co-morbidities which seem to be associated
with greater risk of death (heart disease, diabetes, and respiratory problems) are not high in the school age population.
The *Science* article continued:

Relying on those encouraging if scant data—and the reassuring knowledge that very few children get severely ill from
COVID-19—some governments are beginning to reopen
schools. Denmark sent children up to age [eleven] back on
[April 15], and Germany welcomed back mostly older children on [April 29]. Some Israeli schools reopened on [May
3]; the Netherlands and the Canadian province of Quebec
plan to reopen many primary schools on [May 11]. The steps
are tentative; most schools are resuming with reduced class
sizes, shortened school days, and extra handwashing.[60]

Notice what wasn't in those return-to-school plans: face masks. That's because the medical professionals, looking at the data on schoolchildren, didn't think it made sense.

A recent French study which was highlighted in *Bloomberg News* also found the same pattern that children do not appear to transmit the virus to others, and when children are infected, their symptoms are much less severe.

> School kids don't appear to transmit the new coronavirus to peers or teachers, a French study found, weighing in on the crucial topic of children's role in propagating Covid-19.
>
> Scientists at Institut Pasteur studied 1,340 people in Crepy-en-Valois, a town northeast of Paris that suffered an outbreak in February and March, including 510 students from six primary schools. They found three probable cases among kids that didn't lead to more infections among other pupils or teachers.
>
> The study confirms that children appear to show fewer telltale symptoms than adults and be less contagious, providing a justification for school re-openings in countries from Denmark to Switzerland.[61]

We need to respond to data. The data are showing that children are not at risk for SARS-CoV-2 and we don't need to worry about them transmitting the virus to adults in their lives.

Even an opinion piece from CNN, written by the former executive director of UNICEF, urging a return of children to school, didn't advocate for face masks.

> There are safe ways to do this. School operations will need to align with public health measures, and adjustments will need to be made when there is new information on risks or changes in local transmission and conditions.
>
> There is no denying that a lot needs to be done to increase health safety in schools—especially in the poorest communities. For example, handwashing stations, disinfection and physical distancing.[62]

We want children to be protected, but we also want them to learn and develop.

Practically all Americans have come to know Dr. Anthony Fauci during the COVID-19 epidemic, and most would credit him as exceptionally cautious in his pronouncements. In an interview with CNN in June 2020 he provided some of his thoughts on the reopening of schools and what that might look like:

> The idea of keeping schools closed in the fall because of safety concerns for children might be "a bit of a reach," said Dr. Anthony Fauci, director of the National Institute of Allergy and Infectious Diseases.
>
> In a phone interview with CNN Wednesday, Fauci noted that children tend to have milder symptoms or even no symptoms when they are infected with Covid-19.[63]

Fauci is agreeing with the general scientific observation that children do not seem to be severely impacted by COVID-19, and when they do have the virus, they don't seem to pass it on easily to others. As to what those changes might look like, Fauci said:

> "In some situations, there will be no problem for children to go back to school," he said. "In others, you may need to do some modifications. You know, modifications could be breaking up the class, so you don't have a crowded class-room, maybe half in the morning, half in the afternoon, having children doing alternate schedules. There's a whole bunch of things that one can do . . ."
>
> He suggested that one option is to space out children at every other desk, or every third desk in order to maintain proper social distancing.[64]

But in the article, there's no discussion of children being masked. Again, like the classic Sherlock Holmes story of the dog that didn't bark, why is nobody talking about children wearing masks in school? Especially since they mandate all adults to be masked.

The reason is because it's a foolish idea, just as it's foolish for the general public to be masked. Kids will run around school and exhaust themselves, and they need prodigious amounts of oxygen to keep up their activity levels. Adults need oxygen just as much, and we need our social interactions, walks in the glorious sunlight, exercise, and good, healthy food, as we laugh with our friends in the sunshine.

These are the virtues which will now get us through any challenge.

Points to Remember

1. Human beings need to breathe oxygen and exhale carbon dioxide. Oxygen is 20.9 percent of the air we breathe in, but only 16 percent of what we breathe out. OSHA regulations state that any oxygen-level below 19.5 percent is dangerous. Carbon dioxide is only at 0.04 percent in the atmosphere, but 4 percent of the air we breathe out, a hundred-fold increase. Carbon dioxide toxicity begins when those levels are around 10 percent. Masks lower oxygen levels and raise carbon dioxide levels.
2. SARS-CoV-2 spreads mainly through respiratory droplets from infected individuals who are coughing, hacking, or sneezing and in close, sustained contact with others. It does not appear to spread through regular breathing from people in typical social interactions.
3. Masks have varying degrees of effectiveness, but the more effective they are at blocking air flow, the lower your oxygen levels will be, and the higher the carbon dioxide. Studies have shown that masks raise complaints of shortness of breath, headaches, and dizziness, suggesting lower oxygen and higher carbon dioxide levels.
4. You do not need to be six feet apart from a person *and* wearing a mask. The WHO does not recommend a six-foot distance for social distancing, but only a

three-foot distance. Reputable publications such as *The Lancet* have reported there is "scarce" evidence that masks provide effective protection against respiratory infections.

5. Masks disrupt normal patterns of air flow, leading to pathogens being deposited on chin, cheeks, and near eyes. A small study from South Korea showed that COVID-19 easily passed through several different types of masks.

6. Unless you are close to somebody who is singing or speaking very loudly, such as in a choir, the risk of airborne transmission is very low, especially since it is difficult for coughing people to sing. Super-spreader events have appeared to have taken place only in indoor events and among individuals in prolonged close and intimate contact with each other, singing, or talking loudly. Sunlight is a potent killer of this virus, often destroying it within a few minutes.

7. Nursing homes are dangerous for spreading SARS-CoV-2, as the residents normally have lowered immunity. That lowered immunity makes them most susceptible to developing COVID-19 from exposure to SARS-CoV-2. Consider that 42 percent of Covid-19 cases have come from nursing homes, even though they account for only 0.6 percent of the population. Recent data from several states suggest that number might be substantially higher. Having heart disease, diabetes, or chronic lung disease also increases your chances of disease development from any upper respiratory infection.

8. Masks can become virus traps, leading to increased chances for infection when you touch with your hands. The CDC has abundantly documented how well viruses can remain active on N95 respirator masks, and there is no reason to believe the results wouldn't be the same for other types of masks.

9. There's no such thing as an "asymptomatic" carrier, who has the virus without symptoms for weeks, months, or years. The *New England Journal of Medicine* recently published an article from several researchers claiming that wearing a mask outside of a health care facility "offers little, if any, protection from infection."

10. Children should return to school in the fall without masks. Multiple studies and infection patterns indicate children are less likely to get infected, and when they are infected they have more mild symptoms (and thus are less likely to be coughing and hacking) and do not spread the virus to teachers, parents, or grandparents.

Final Thoughts

Scientific understanding is a continuing process. What we have put together in this book is intended as part of a continuing dialogue on how to best respond to the SARS-Cov-2 infection and the development of COVID-19. We expect many more things are to be learned about this outbreak. Even at this point there are many things which are unclear, such as whether this virus was the result of a natural spillover from bats who lived several hundreds of miles from Wuhan, China, or released from a lab in Wuhan.

One of the latest claims is that SARS-CoV-2 is altering the immune function of those who contract it.[65] This is an unusual occurrence for a typical corona virus, but common for retroviruses like HIV, supporting the contention this is a laboratory created virus. Several researchers have noted HIV sequences in SARS-CoV-2. This is not unexpected when the bat viruses were grown in Vero monkey kidney cells. This continuously growing cell line contains many monkey viruses including SIV. SIV is the closest ancestor to HIV. How else do you get sequences from a monkey virus in a bat virus? The most likely scenario is the common laboratory practice of passaging viruses through cell lines of different species in order to adapt them to infect the cells without killing them in what is commonly referred to as "gain of function" research. We have experienced several deadly pandemics over the past four decades of my career. All clearly started from these laboratory practices, despite the best efforts of the majority of virology experts to prohibit gain of function research. That COVID-19 is a man-made disaster, a plague of corruption is a pox on all of our houses. Our response must not result in more suffering and loss of life than the virus/disease. Such is the case of universal mask use as we have made a strong case that not only do the masks not prevent spread of SARS-CoV-2, they do not ameliorate COVID-19. Based on our fair and balanced interpretation of the data we can only conclude that the masks are doing more damage, particularly to the most vulnerable to developing COVID-19 from a SARS-CoV-2 infection. As an alumna of the University of Virginia, I quote its founder Thomas Jefferson: "[T]his institution will be based on the illimitable freedom of the human mind. For here we are not afraid to follow the truth wherever it may lead, nor tolerate error so long as reason is left free to combat it." It's time to restore freedom and reason to all Americans.

Endnotes

1   "Earth's Atmosphere Composition: Nitrogen, Oxygen, Argon and CO_2," *Earth How*, accessed June 15, 2020, www.earthhow.com/earth-atmosphere-composition/.

2   Ibid.

3   Ibid.

4   "What Are the Normal Oxygen Levels in Humans?" *Reference.com*, accessed June 15, 2020, www.reference.com/world-view/normal-oxygen-levels-humans-602ffe726c4b8107.

5   Sean Kane, "Here's the Longest People Have Survived Without Air, Food, Water, Sunshine, or Sleep," *Science Alert*, last modified June 10, 2016, accessed June 15, 2020, www.sciencealert.com/here-s-the-longest-people-have-survived-without-air-food-water-sunshine-or-sleep.

6   "What Gases Do Humans Exhale?" *Reference.com*, accessed June 15, 2020, www.reference.com/science/gases-humans-exhale-2e229a37e5894295.

7   "Respiratory Protection," Occupational Health and Safety Administration, accessed June 25, 2020, https://www.osha.gov/sites/default/files/2019-03/respiratoryprotection.pdf.

8   Claire Gillespie, "Does Wearing a Face Mask Reduce Oxygen—and Can It Increase CO_2 Levels? Here's What Experts Say," *Health.com*, last modified May 13, 2020, accessed June 15, 2020, www.health.com/condition/infectious-diseases/coronavirus/does-wearing-face-mask-increase-co2-levels.

9   Ibid.

10 Ibid.

[11] Antonio Lazzarino, A. Steptoe, M. Hamer, & S. Michie, "Covid-19: Important Potential Side Effects of Wearing Masks that We Should Bear in Mind," *British Medical Journal*, 2020; 369:m1435 (April 9, 2020): doi: 10.1136/bmj.m1435.

[12] Ibid.

[13] Ibid.

[14] "Guidance on Preparing Workplaces for COVID-19," U.S. Department of Labor, Occupational Safety and Health Administration, accessed June 17, 2020, www.osha.gov/Publications/OSHA3990.pdf.

[15] Ibid. at p. 5.

[16] Joshua Bote, "The CDC Says Coronavirus 'Does Not Spread Easily' on Surfaces or Objects. Here's What We Know," *USA Today*, May 21, 2020, updated May 27, 2020, www.usatoday.com/story/news/health/2020/05/21/coronavirus-news-what-cdc-saying-covid-19-surfaces/5235317002/.

[17] Ibid.

[18] Mayo Clinic Staff, "COVID-19: How Much Protection Do Face Masks Offer?" Mayo Clinic, accessed June 17, 2020, www.mayoclinic.org/diseases-conditions/coronavirus/in-depth/coronavirus-mask/art-20485449

[19] Ibid.

[20] Ibid.

[21] Ibid.

[22] Terri Rebmann, Ruth Carrico, & Jing Wang, "Physiologic and Other Effects and Compliance with Long-Term Respirator Use Among Medical Intensive Care Unit Nurses," *American Journal of Infection Control*, Vol. 41 (12), p. 1218-1223: doi:10.1016/j.ajic.2013.02.017.

[23] John W. Cherrie, Andrew Apsley, Hilary Cowie, Susanne Steinle, William Mueller, Chun Lin, Claire J. Horwell, Anne Sleeuwenhoek, & Miranda Loh, "Effectiveness of Face Masks Used to Protect Beijing Residents Against Particulate Air Pollution," *Journal of Occupational and Environmental Medicine*, Vol. 75(6): 446-452, April 9, 2018: doi: 10.1136/oemed-2017-104765.

[24] Shuo Feng, Chen Shen, Nan Xia, Wei Song, & Benjamin J. Cowling, "Rational Use of Face Mask Use in the COVID-19 Pandemic," *The*

Lancet, Vol. 8, issue 5, p.434-436 (May 1, 2020), doi: 10.1016/ S2213-2600(20)30134-X.

25 Ibid.

26 Ibid.

27 Ibid.

28 Ibid.

29 Ibid.

30 Elda Bastian, "The Face Mask Debate Reveals a Scientific Double Standard," *Wired*, April 8, 2020, www.wired.com/story/the-face-mask-debate-reveals-a-scientific-double-standard/.

31 Ibid.

32 Ibid.

33 I.M. Viola, et al., "Face Coverings, Aerosol Dispersion and Mitigation of Virus Transmission Risk," May 19, 2020, *arXiv*, www.arvix.org/ abs/2005.10720.

34 Russell Blaylock, "Face Masks Pose Serious Risks to the Healthy," Green Med Info, May 16, 2020, www.greenmedinfo.com/blog/dr-blaylock-face-masks-pose-serious-risks-healthy11.

35 Ibid.

36 Molly Walker, "Study: Masks Fail to Filter Virus in Coughing COVID-19 Patients," *Medpage Today*, April 6, 2020, www.medpagetoday.com/infectiousdisease/covid19/85814.

37 Jeremy Hammond, "New York Times Laughably Lies that the Mask Debate is Settled," *Jeremy R. Hammond*, accessed June 8, 2020, https://www.jeremyrhammond.com/2020/06/05/new-york-times-laughably-lies-that-the-mask-debate-is-settled/.

38 Kai Kupferschmidt, "Why Do Some COVID-19 Patients Infect Many Others, Whereas Most Don't Spread the Virus at All?" *Science*, May 19, 2020, accessed June 21, 2020, https://www.sciencemag.org/ news/2020/05/why-do-some-covid-19-patients-infect-many-others-whereas-most-don-t-spread-virus-all.

39 Ibid.

40 Ibid.

41 "Sunlight Destroys Coronavirus Quickly, Say U.S. Scientists," Medical Express, April 24, 2020, accessed June 25, 2020, www.medicalxpress.com/news/2020-04-sunlight-coronavirus-quickly-scientists.html.

[42] Kai Kupferschmidt, "Why Do Some COVID-19 Patients Infect Many Others, Whereas Most Don't Spread the Virus at All?" *Science*, May 19, 2020, accessed June 21, 2020, https://www.sciencemag.org/news/2020/05/why-do-some-covid-19-patients-infect-many-others-whereas-most-don-t-spread-virus-all.

[43] Avik Roy, "The Most Important Coronavirus Statistic: 42% of U.S. Deaths Are From 0.6% of the Population," Forbes, May 26, 2020, www.forbes.com/sites/theapothecary/2020/05/26/nursing-homes-assisted-living-facilities-0-6-of-the-u-s-population-43-of-u-s-covid-19-deaths/#5d62d2bc74cd.

[44] Ibid.

[45] Ibid.

[46] Niall MCarthy, "COVID-19 Patients with Existing Conditions Far More Likely to Die," *Statista*, June 16, 2020, www.statista.com/chart/22018/coronavirus-pre-existing-conditions/.

[47] Ibid.

[48] "New Surgical Mask Doesn't Just Trap Viruses, It Renders Them Harmless," *Science Daily*, January 5, 2017, www.sciencedaily.com/releases/2017/01/170105160228.htm.

[49] "Recommended Guidance for Extended Use and Limited Reuse of N95 Filtering Facepiece Respirators in Healthcare Settings," *Centers for Disease Control, National Institute for Occupational Safety and Health*, last reviewed March 27, 2020, accessed June 16, 2020, www.cdc.gov/niosh/topics/hcwcontrols/recommendedguidanceextuse.html.

[50] Ibid.

[51] Hillary Brueck, "The WHO Said Asymptomatic Transmission is 'Very Rare,' then Said That Was a 'Misunderstanding.' Here's What You Need to Know," *Business Insider*, June 9, 2020, www.businessinsider.com/who-clarifies-comment-that-asymptomatic-transmission-is-very-rare-2020-6.

[52] Ibid.

[53] Ibid.

[54] Kenji Mizumoto, Katsuchi Kagaya, Alexander Zarebski, and Gerardo Chowell, "Estimating the Asymptomatic Proportion of Coronavirus Disease 2019 (COVID-19) Cases on Board the Diamond Princess

Cruise Ship, Yokohama, Japan, 2020," *European Surveillance*, Rapid Communication, (March 12, 2020) doi: 10.2807/1560-7917.

55   Michael Klompas, Charles Morris, Julia Sinclair, Madelyn Pearson & Erica Shenoy, "Universal Masking in Hospitals in the Covid-19 Era," *New England Journal of Medicine*, vol. 382: e63, (May 2020) : doi: 10.1056/NEJMp2006372.

56   Sam Dorman, "Joy Behar Says She and Her Husband Drive Around Looking for People Not Wearing Masks," *Fox News*, June 23, 2020, www.foxnews.com/media/joy-behar-husband-drive-no-masks.

57   Ibid.

58   Helen Branswel, "How Likely Are Kids to Get Covid-19? Scientists See a 'Huge Puzzle' Without Easy Answers," STAT News, June 18, 2020, www.statnews.com/2020/06/18/how-likely-are-kids-to-get-covid-19-scientists-see-a-huge-puzzle-without-easy-answers/.

59   Gretchen Vogel & Jennifer Couzin-Frankel, "Should Schools Reopen? Kids' Role in Pandemic Still a Mystery," *Science* magazine, May 4, 2020, www.sciencemag.org/news/2020/05/should-schools-reopen-kids-role-pandemic-still-mystery.

60   Ibid.

61   Martha Fourcade, "School Children Don't Spread Coronavirus, French Study Shows," Bloomberg News, June 23, 2020, www.bloomberg.com/news/articles/2020-06-23/school-children-don-t-spread-coronavirus-french-study-shows.

62   Henrietta Fore, "It's Time to Reopen Schools, CNN, June 19, 2020, www.cnn.com/2020/06/19/opinions/time-to-reopen-schools-covid-19-fore/index.html.

63   Annie Grayer, "Fauci Says It's Time to Think About Re-Opening Schools," CNN, June 4, 2020, www.cnn.com/2020/06/03/us/fauci-schools-reopening-coronavirus/index.html.

64   Ibid.

65   Gina Kolata, "How the Coronavirus Short-Circuits the Immune System," *New York Times*, June 26, 2020, www.nytimes.com/2020/06/26/health/coronavirus-immune-system.html.

Acknowledgments

I'd first like to thank my wonderful partner in life, Linda, and our two children, Jacqueline and Ben for their constant love and support. I'd also like to thank my mother, Josephine, and my father, Jack, for always encouraging me. I have the best brother in the world, Jay, and am appreciative to his wife, Andrea, and their three kids, Anna, John, and Laura.

I've been fortunate to have some of the greatest teachers in the world, Paul Rago, Elizabeth White, Ed Balsdon, Brother Richard Orona, Clinton Bond, Robert Haas, Carol Lashoff, David Alvarez, Giancarlo Trevisan, Bernie Segal, James Frey, Donna Levin, and James Dalessandro.

Thanks to the fantastic friends of my life, John Wible, John Henry, Pete Klenow, Chris Sweeney, Suzanne Golibart, Gina Cioffi Loud, Eric Holm, Susanne Brown, Rick Friedling, Max Swafford, Sherilyn Todd, Rick and Robin Kreutzer, Christie and Joaquim Perreira, and Tricia Mangiapane.

Lastly, I'd like to thank my agent, Johanna Maaghul, and at Skyhorse the fabulous Caroline Russomanno and Hector Carosso, and for the faith shown in me over the years by publisher Tony Lyons.